FIT TO FLY

A Guide to Healthy Weight Loss

CHARITY SAGO

CONTENTS

DEDICATION

This book is dedicated to God Almighty for the gift of the Holy Spirit which has been of tremendous help.

I also dedicate this book to my parents (Mr & Mrs Sago) and my siblings. I love you all.

ACKNOWLEDGMENT

I appreciate God Almighty for being intentional about me and for His unending love and support.

1. BASIC TERMS DESCRIPTION

What is Weight?

The Oxford Dictionary defines weight as a body's relative mass or the amount of matter it contains that causes a downward force; the weight of an individual or thing.

Essentially, weight alludes to how weighty an item or an individual is.

Body weight is maintained by how much energy that an individual gets from food utilization and how much energy that is spent while playing out his day-to-day exercises.

What is Weight Loss?

Weight Loss is a lessening in body weight which can be brought about by either following an eating regimen, working out, falling wiped out, or going through a few distressing circumstances.

What is Health?

As indicated by the World Wellbeing Association (WHO), health is a condition of complete physical, mental, and social prosperity and not simply the shortfall of illness or sickness. This suggests that wholeness is the state of health.

Kinds of Heath

There are various kinds of health, going from physical health to spiritual health, to mental health, to financial health, etc. In any case, physical fitness and mental health are the most examined kinds of health.

Physical Health: The normal function of the body is what we mean when we talk about physical health.

Actual wellbeing isn't simply the shortfall of sickness. Numerous aspects of life are related to physical health, such as: resting soundly, eating adjusted consumes less calories, doing works out, great cleanliness, and resting great. Such viewpoints can be assembled into three principal parts of actual wellbeing. The three primary parts are rest and rest, sustenance (adjusted diet), and actual work (development and exercise).

Legitimate consideration of actual wellbeing assists with decreasing the gamble of ailment or illness. A person with sound actual wellbeing will appreciate smooth working cycles of the body framework.

Mental Health: Emotional wellness alludes to an individual's personal, social, and mental prosperity. Psychological wellness is likewise all around as significant as actual wellbeing. A person with poor psychological wellness is probably going to incur hurt for his actual wellbeing. To live a full and active life, a person must have good mental health.

Spiritual Health: The quality of a person's connection to a higher power is the focus of spiritual health. It demonstrates a person's capacity to have faith in a higher power, to discover his purpose in his relationship with that power, and to experience peace of mind in that relationship.

Because a person has faith in the abilities of the higher power, good spiritual health produces confidence and peace.

Financial Health: As indicated by the Financial Health Network, financial health is a composite estimation of a person's monetary life. Monetary wellbeing manages how an individual spends, saves, acquires, and designs.

Financial health just shows an individual's strength in his\her funds. Great monetary wellbeing shows an individual's capacity to ingest shocks from monetary misfortune and endeavor to accomplish his/her monetary objectives.

Great monetary wellbeing prompts less concerns. Individuals with better monetary wellbeing will have rest due to the trust in their capacities to routinely address their issues.

What is Healthy Weight Loss?

Healthy Weight Loss is a demonstration of shedding pounds continuously by following a way of life that includes following good dieting designs, standard actual work, and overseeing unpleasant circumstances.

Individuals who follow a slow course of getting in shape are bound to have sound weight reduction than individuals who rapidly get more fit.

2. WHY LOSE WEIGHT?

There are several reasons why a person can decide to lose weight. But it is important to note the benefits of losing weight in a healthy way. Some of the benefits of healthy weight loss include;

- **Improved Health of the Heart:** Your heart is

  an area of strength that upholds the course of oxygen-rich blood to every one of the organs and tissues all through your body. Conveying additional body weight puts extra weight on your heart and may harm the muscle, which can increase your chances of cardiovascular breakdown.

  Shedding pounds in a solid manner assists with further developing the heart capabilities. Being overweight makes your heart work harder to move blood through the body. Shedding some weight lessens tension on your conduits and weight on your heart.

- **Better Immune System**: The immune system

  is put to a lot of strain by excess weight. This prompts more colds and different diseases. The immune system is strengthened, and overall health is improved when people lose weight.

- **Reduced Risk of Diabetes:** You are multiple times bound to foster diabetes on the off chance that you're overweight than if you are at a normal weight.

  Diabetes is a long-term condition that can make you more likely to get kidney disease, neuropathy, heart disease, and other serious health problems. Getting more fit brings down the glucose in the body which brings down the gamble of diabetes.

- **Eased Movement**: Every aspect of life is impacted by the benefits of weight loss. Development becomes simpler for a person with sound weight. Everyday exercises like sitting, standing, going up the steps, running, strolling, and so on are more straightforward with less weight.

- **Less Perspiration:** Hugging people is less embarrassing when they are carrying less weight because the body sweats less.

- **Less Joint Pains**: Less weight implies less
  pressure and aggravation in the knees, elbows,
  and hips.

- **Lowered Risk of Stroke**: Advancing toward
  your objective weight brings down your stroke
  risk. Shedding pounds diminishes the stress on
  your heart as well as decreases the strain on
  your veins, making it doubtful that a blood
  coagulation will create.

- **Lowered Risk of Cancer**: Weight reduction
  brings down the gamble of explicit tumors. As
  your weight drops, so does your gamble of
  illnesses like pancreatic, kidney, bosom (in
  ladies past menopause), endometrial, and liver
  disease.

- **Less Stress:** Food varieties with a high fat,
  sugar, and salt substance - particularly handled
  carbs - can set off elevated degrees of cortisol
  otherwise known as. the pressure chemical. A
  solid weight reduction routine can switch this.

- **Balanced Mood:** At a moderate weight, the

thyroid can work more effectively which advances adjusted chemicals. Additionally, exercising while trying to lose weight causes the brain to release endorphins (feel-good chemicals) resulting in a more positive attitude and balanced mood.

- **Improved Mobility:** Your knees and other joints

will benefit from losing weight. Indeed, even insignificant weight decrease lessens joint agony and makes it simpler to move around.

That improvement might make you more leaned to work out, which proceeds with the descending pattern in your weight and the vertical pattern in your wellness.

- **Improved Sleep:** Weight reduction further

develops rest and lifts energy. Sleep apnea frequently affects overweight individuals. It is a condition where fat stores in the neck make it harder to inhale, which brings about regular renewals over the course of the evening. Shedding pounds may not wipe out the issue, however it can altogether further develop rest quality.

After getting in shape, individuals will generally rest all through the whole evening and experience better of rest. You will have more energy throughout the day as a result.

- **Increased Energy:** Conveying additional

  weight requires the body to utilize a great deal of energy. At the point when somebody sheds pounds, their energy levels will soar. Besides, the body can work much better when it is provided with nutritious food.

  It is possible that giving one's body the right vitamins and minerals can also make it easier to think, making work seem less overwhelming.

- **Increased Sexual Desire:** Shedding pounds

  can build your sex drive. It can give an individual a stronger sexual desire. Hormonal changes from weight reduction can expand your drive.

- **Improved Sense of Taste:** Getting in shape

  can work on your feeling of taste. It's not satisfactory why, yet individuals who get thinner frequently report that it hones their feeling of taste. Thus, you might find that you can diminish segment sizes yet get a similar happiness from a feast.

- **Expanded Confidence:** The advantages of

  weight reduction go significantly farther than just superior cardiovascular wellbeing. As a matter of fact, getting more fit can emphatically affect practically every part of an individual's life.

  Most of the time, when people decide to lose weight, they feel better about themselves. This equivalent regard converts into different connections.
  Gaining ground can work on your confidence. Not every one of the advantages of weight reduction are physical. Changes in the way you feel about yourself are also vital and worth seeing and celebrating.

- **Improved Sensitivity to Insulin:** When people

  with type 2 diabetes start losing weight, they typically become more sensitive to insulin. That is on the grounds that an abundance of muscle to fat ratio causes irritation that antagonistically influences how insulin (the chemical that controls glucose) capabilities. Even if you only lose a little bit of weight, you might start to see results.

- **Adventure Begins:** Getting thinner is a troublesome errand. To maintain their adventurous spirit, people who lose weight may feel compelled to try new things they would never have thought of before.

  Weight loss isn't just good for your health in the physical sense. Shedding pounds opens another universe of exercises that were beforehand inconceivable: entertainment meccas, thrill rides, swimming, climbing, and so on.

  Shedding pounds likewise frees the person up to a gutsy universe of various healthy eating regimens. Adjusting a solid eating regimen requires cooking. As individuals shed pounds, they'll learn new recipes and evaluate new procedures in the kitchen.

- **Improved Memory:** The cerebrum requires satisfactory nutrients and minerals to work. At the point when individuals get more fit, they will generally devour better food sources with higher cell reinforcement levels bringing about superior memory abilities.

- **Reduced Need for Medications:** Reduced use

of medications is a sign of better overall health. Consequently, having healthy weight prompts decreased need for medications which in turn prompts better overall health.

3. WRONG CONCEPTS OF WEIGHT LOSS

There are several misconceptions about weight loss. People have adopted their own theories of weight loss. In your research for tips on weight loss, you may have come across some of these misconceptions. Many concepts of weight loss are false. Some of the wrong concepts of weight loss are explained below.

1. All Calories are Equivalent: The calorie is an estimation of energy. All calories have a similar energy content. In any case, this does not imply that all calorie sources affect your weight. Various food sources go through various metabolic pathways and can affect hunger and the chemicals that control your body weight. For instance, a protein calorie is not equivalent to a fat or carb calorie.

Not all calorie sources meaningfully affect your wellbeing and weight. For instance, protein can increase digestion, decrease hunger, and work on the capability of weight-managing chemicals. Consequently, supplanting carbs and fat with protein can support your digestion and diminish hunger and desires, all while upgrading the capability of some weight-controlling chemicals.

Additionally, calories from entire food sources like natural products will quite often be significantly more filling than calories from refined food sources, like treats.

2. Shedding Pounds is a Direct Interaction:

Contrary to popular belief, losing weight typically is not a one-way street. Getting thinner can consume a large chunk of the day and the cycle is for the most part not straight, as your weight will in general change all over by limited quantities. You might lose weight on some days and weeks, but you might gain a little on others. This is not a reason to worry.

It is normal for people to lose or gain a few pounds in weight. For instance, you might be conveying more food in your stomach related framework or clutching more water than expected. This is much more articulated in ladies, as water weight can vary altogether during the feminine cycle.

However long the general pattern is going downwards, regardless of the amount it changes, you will in any case prevail with regards to shedding pounds over the long haul.

3. Weight Loss can be aided by Supplements: The weight reduction supplement industry is gigantic. Different organizations guarantee that their enhancements make sensational impacts, however they are seldom extremely powerful when considered.

The principal reason that enhancements work for certain individuals is a self-influenced consequence. Individuals succumb to the advertising strategies and believe the enhancements should assist them with getting thinner, so they become more aware of what they eat. Most enhancements for weight reduction are incapable. All that ones can assist you with losing a touch of weight, probably.

4. Weight is about Determination: It is erroneous to say that your weight is about self-discipline. Heftiness can be a consequence of such countless contributing elements. Various hereditary factors are related with corpulence, and different ailments like hypothyroidism can increase your chances of weight gain.

Your body additionally has various chemicals and natural pathways that should direct body weight. These will generally be useless in individuals with heftiness, making it a lot harder to get in shape and keep it off.

Attempting to apply determination and deliberately eating less notwithstanding the leptin-driven starvation signal is unimaginably troublesome. Obviously, this doesn't imply that individuals ought to surrender and acknowledge their hereditary destiny. Getting healthy weight is achievable.

It is essential to keep in mind that obesity is a very complicated condition. There are numerous hereditary, natural, and ecological elements that influence body weight. All things considered, shedding pounds isn't just about self-control.

5. Exercise More and Eat Less: Simply put, body fat is stored energy. To lose fat, you really want to consume a bigger number of calories than you take in. Therefore, it appears to be just sensible that eating less and moving more would cause weight reduction.

While this guidance works in principle, particularly if you make a long-lasting way of life change, it is a terrible proposal for those with a serious weight issue.

A great many people who heed this guidance wind up recovering any shed pounds because of physiological and biochemical elements. Teaching somebody with corpulence to just eat less and move more resembles advising somebody with melancholy to encourage or somebody with liquor abuse to drink less. Advising individuals with weight issues to simply eat less and move more is inadequate counsel that seldom works in the long haul.

Diet and exercise alone will not help you lose weight unless you make a significant and ongoing shift in your mindset and behavior. Limiting your food admission and it isn't sufficient to get more actual work.

6. You get fat from Carbs: Low-carb diets can help weight reduction. By and large, this happens even without cognizant calorie limitation. You will lose weight if you eat a lot of protein and little carbs.

All things considered; this does not imply that carbs cause weight gain. As a matter of fact, entire food varieties that are high in carbs are exceptionally solid. Yet, it is additionally vital to take note of that refined carbs like refined grains and sugar are certainly connected to weight gain.

7. Fat makes you Fat: The obesity epidemic has frequently been attributed to fat. Fat is very calorie-thick and typical in low quality foods. While it adds to your complete calorie consumption, fat alone doesn't cause weight gain.

Also, consumes less calories that are high in fat however low in carbs have been displayed to cause weight reduction in various examinations.

Although consuming unhealthy, high-calorie, fat-laden

junk food will unquestionably make you fat, this macronutrient is not the only culprit. Your body needs solid fats to work appropriately, as a matter of fact.

8. Losing weight necessitates skipping Breakfast: Concentrates on show that morning meal captains will generally weigh more than breakfast eaters. Nonetheless, this is presumably because individuals who have breakfast are bound to have other sound way of life propensities.

9. Fast Food is continuously stuffing: Not all fast food is undesirable. Considering individuals' expanded wellbeing awareness, many food chains have begun offering better choices. It is feasible to get meals that are healthy at considered eateries. Most modest drive-through eateries frequently give better options in contrast to their fundamental contributions. These food sources may not fulfill the requests of every wellbeing cognizant individual; however, they are yet a fair decision on the off chance that you don't have the opportunity or energy to prepare a good dinner.

10. Diet Foods can aid in weight loss: A great deal of unhealthy food is promoted as sound. Low-fat, fat-free, processed gluten-free foods, as well as beverages high in sugar, are examples. You ought to have one or two doubts of any wellbeing claims on food bundling, particularly on handled things.

 The weight reduction industry believes you should accept that diets work. Notwithstanding, concentrates on show that counting calories seldom works in the long haul. Individuals who diet are probably going to put on weight from here on out. In this manner, slimming down is a great investment for weight gain in the future!

Truly, you most likely shouldn't move toward weight reduction with an eating less junk food outlook. Regardless of what the weight reduction industry would have you accept, counting calories normally doesn't work. All things considered, make it an objective to change your way of life for all time and become a better, more joyful, and physically fit individual.

11. **Obese People are Unhealthy and Slim People are Sound:** This is not true. A few slim individuals have equivalent persistent sicknesses that are common in obese people. The main consideration is where your fat develops. If you have a ton of fat in your stomach region, you are at a more serious gamble of metabolic sickness.

12. Eat Too Little: Decreasing calories however much as could be expected can appear to be an extraordinary method for getting thinner, yet it can blow up. If you don't eat enough, you will be more open to outside influences and more likely to make unhealthy food choices that will not help you achieve your goals.

Eating too little won't work in the long haul. That absence of energy and consistent appetite from your super quick bites can likewise make it harder to get spurred to work out. Losing more than two pounds in seven days implies you are likely not eating enough.

13. Sipping your Liquid Calories: Fluids don't fight off the satisfaction yearn for long. However, eating solid food sources do. Heavy liquid sipping can make way for weight gain. The sippers can end up consuming additional 400 calories over the course of the day.

14. Not getting enough Sleep: At the point when life gets going, rest is many times the principal thing to give up. Apart from its effect on mental health and emotional health, not getting sufficient closed eye raises the gamble for weight gain.

Hormones that control hunger and fullness change when people don't get enough sleep. It is good to get an average of seven to eight hours of closed eye every evening. Because it has been linked to better health, such as a lower risk of heart disease, diabetes, obesity, and depression.

15. Skipping Protein: It is not ideal to skip protein in your meals. Why skip protein in breakfast and lunch? Protein is more satisfying. It takes more time to process, so you feel fuller for longer. One of the most incredible ways to deal with protein is to eat it over the course of the day.

16. Decreasing your Portion Sizes: At the point when individuals are served more food, they will quite often eat more. Along your weight reduction venture, measure your parts to sort out precisely the amount you are eating.

17. Reducing Intake of Water: Water consumption has been linked to weight loss in some studies, but there is no conclusive evidence to support this claim. A definite truth is that water assists you with remaining hydrated for zero calories and zero sugar. It is very healthy to trade water for soft drinks as it can cut many calories from your everyday count. The general rule of drinking water is to drink enough to make your urine pale yellow.

18. Nibbling Carelessly: Indeed, a tidbit can add nourishment to your eating routine. Additionally, they can alleviate hunger, preventing overeating at subsequent meals. Yet, occasionally, we nibble out of fatigue, or end up getting such many calories from brushing. Have a plan for snacks to avoid overeating. Snacks should be three to four hours after a meal, and they should be satisfying. Snacks that contain both protein and fiber should be considered.

19. Having a Win Big or Bust Attitude: Although perfection-or-bust thinking is common, it can hinder your efforts to lose weight.

If you commit an error on your journey to healthy weight loss, don't feel embarrassed. Rather than feeling ashamed, pause for a minute to thoroughly consider what occurred with no judgment. You might understand that you rashly added an unhealthy treat to your menu.

20. Knocking Exercise off your Daily Agenda:
Indeed, life occurs and at times that implies exercise
plans don't work out. But focusing on active work is
great. It is one of the best indicators of long-term
weight maintenance, according to research.

Go for a bicycle ride, walk the dog down the street,
swim, have a dance party, or do reinforcing moves
while you cook. You can likewise split it up into brief
sessions over the course of your day.

4. HEALTHY METHODS FOR LOSING WEIGHT

Many diets, supplements, and meal replacement plans promise quick weight loss, but there is no scientific evidence to support their claims. However, there are some scientific approaches to weight management that are beneficial to health. Some of such healthy approaches are composed underneath.

✔ **Intermittent Fasting:** Intermittent fasting (IF) is an example of eating that involves fasting for a stipulated period and eating within a limited time span during the fasting.

Some examples of intermittent fasting include substitute day fasting (that is eat less calories on fasting days and eat adequate calories on non-fasting day), the 5:2 eating style (that is fast on two days of the week and eat 500–600 calories on days of fasting), and the 16/8 style (fast for 16 hours and eat just during an 8-hour window).

It is important to note that it is ideal to embrace a good dieting design on non-fasting days and to abstain from over-eating.

✔ **Tracking Your Diet and Exercise:** To get in

shape, you ought to know what you eat and drink every day. Keeping track of these things in a journal or an online food tracker is one way to accomplish this. Following a well-crafted plan for meals and exercise might be useful for weight reduction since it increases inspiration.

✔ **Eating Carefully:** Careful eating is a training

where individuals focus on how and where they eat food. This training can empower individuals to partake in the food they eat and may assist with advancing weight reduction.

 As people are frequently busy, they are more likely to eat rapidly on the run, in the vehicle, working at their work areas, and sitting in front of the television. Thus, many individuals are scarcely mindful of the food they are eating.

Strategies for careful eating include careful selection of healthy meals, eating while seated at a dining table, paying attention to the food and enjoying the experience, avoiding interruptions while eating, eating slowly.

✔ **Including Protein in Meals:** Protein can control hunger chemicals to assist with feeling full. A meal that contains high protein can keep a person going for a few hours. It would be nice to include eggs, oats, nuts, etc in your meals.

✔ **Reduced Intake of Sugar and Refined Carbohydrate:** Refined grains go through handling to eliminate the wheat and the microbe, which contain a large portion of the grain's fiber and supplements. White bread, white rice, and regular pasta are examples of these. These food varieties rush to process, and they convert to glucose quickly. Overabundance glucose enters the blood and incites the chemical insulin, which advances fat capacity in the fat tissue. This adds to weight gain.

Whole grains are more likely to satisfy hunger and make you feel fuller, which could help you eat fewer calories. Great food trades include entire grain rice, bread, and pasta rather than the white renditions, organic product, nuts, and seeds rather than high sugar snacks, spice teas and organic product implanted water rather than high sugar soft drinks, and smoothies with water or milk rather than natural product juice.

✔ **Eating a lot of Fiber:** Contrary to sugar and

starch, which can be broken down in the small intestine, plant-based carbohydrates are referred to as dietary fiber. Consuming a lot of fiber can make you feel fuller longer, which could help you lose weight. Fiber-rich food varieties include entire grain breakfast cereals, entire wheat pasta, entire grain bread, oats, rye, leafy foods, peas, beans, nuts, and seeds.

✔ **Adjusting Stomach Microorganisms:**

Everyone has various sorts and measures of microscopic organisms in their stomachs. A few kinds might expand how much energy the individual concentrates from food, prompting fat statement and weight gain while certain food sources can build the quantity of good microorganisms in the stomach.

A portion of the food sources can build the quantity of good microscopic organisms in the stomach incorporate vegetables and other plant-based food varieties, prebiotic food sources, matured food sources like yogurt and kimchi, and so forth.

✔ **Getting a Decent Night's Rest:** Research

proposes that deficient or low-quality rest dials back the cycle in which the body switches calories over completely to energy, called digestion. At the point when digestion is less viable, the body might store unused energy as fat.

Poor sleep can also lead to insulin resistance and elevated cortisol levels, which in turn encourage fat storage.

✔ **Taking Control of your Stress:** As part of the

body's fight or flight response, stress causes the release of hormones like adrenaline and cortisol, which initially reduce appetite. Nonetheless, when individuals are under consistent pressure, cortisol can stay in the circulation system for longer, which will build their craving and possibly lead to them eating more.

Cortisol flags the need to renew the body's dietary stores from the favored wellspring of fuel, carb. Insulin then, at that point, moves the sugar from carbs from the blood to the muscles and cerebrum. If the individual doesn't involve

this sugar in survival, the body will store it as
fat.

A few techniques for controlling stress-level and
relieving stress include yoga, meditation,
breathing and unwinding strategies, swimming,
strolling, etc.

5. MAINTAINING A HEALTHY WEIGHT LOSS

Losing too much weight too quickly could make you more likely to get certain health problems, like gallstones, or problems that come with bad dieting, like not drinking enough water or not getting enough nutrients, happen. It is possible that people who lose weight quickly will gain it back in the future. It is suggested that individuals should aim for a healthy weight reduction of around 1-2 pounds each week.

It is vital to recall that there are no convenient solutions with regards to weight reduction. The most ideal way to oversee weight is to eat a nutritious, adjusted diet. This ought to incorporate 10 parts of leafy foods, great quality protein, and entire grains. It is additionally helpful to exercise consistently for an average of 30 minutes daily.

While getting in shape is hard for some individuals, it is considerably challenging to keep being in shape. The vast majority who lose a lot of weight have regained it 2 to 3 years after the fact. One hypothesis about recovering shed pounds is that individuals who decline how much calories they consume to get thinner experience a drop in the rate their bodies consume calories. This makes it progressively challenging to get in shape over time.

A lower pace of consuming calories may likewise make it simpler to recover weight after a more typical healthy eating regimen is continued. Consequently, it is not advisable to go on incredibly low-calorie diets and fast weight reduction.

Healthy weight reduction has medical advantages. It incorporates lower cholesterol and glucose levels, lower pulse, less weight on bones and joints, and less work for the heart. It is imperative to keep up with weight reduction to get medical advantages over a long period.

Weight reduction objectives are arrived at by a blend of changes in diet, dietary patterns, and exercise. When it comes to maintaining a healthy weight, some of the same tactics that work for weight loss also work for weight gain.

When the ideal weight has been reached, extra calories of good food varieties might be added to the everyday eating regimen until the individual attains the right equilibrium of calories to keep up with the ideal weight still up in the air. It might require some investment and record keeping to decide how changing food admission and exercise levels influence weight. A nutritionist can assist with this.

Maintaining weight necessitates continuing to employ behavioral strategies. Know about eating as a reaction to push. Likewise, use exercise, action, or contemplation to adapt as opposed to eating.

Failure does not result from a brief return to previous routines. Focusing on dietary decisions and exercise can assist with keeping up with weight reduction. Recognizing circumstances, like pessimistic states of mind and relational troubles, and utilizing elective strategies for adapting to such circumstances instead of eating can forestall getting back to old propensities.

Exercise is beneficial to everyone, including older people. Ensure that you engage in 30 minutes of real exercise that gets you sweaty. If you can't meet the objective immediately, attempt to exercise at least three times a week. While you are beginning with workout, attempt to consistently move your body. Then, increase the time span you exercise or add another great movement. It is important to chat with your doctor prior to beginning a new or more overwhelming activity program.

For older people at each weight, maturing is related with muscle misfortune, which makes specific exercises troublesome. Being dynamic can assist older people with keeping up with bulk and make it simpler to lead day to day exercises. Older people can take a stroll around the house.

REFERENCES

1. Weight Loss
https://www.topdoctors.co.uk/medical-dictionary
/weight-loss

2. What is good health?

https://www.medicalnewstoday.com/articles/150
998

3. Physical Health | Definition, Examples &
Aspects

https://study.com/learn/lesson/what-is-physical-
health.html

4. What is physical health?
https://health.nzdf.mil.nz/your-health/body/physi
cal-health-and-fitness/what-is-physical-health/

5. What is Financial Health?
   https://finhealthnetwork.org/about/what-is-financ
   ial-health/

6. 9 health benefits of weight loss
   https://www.baptisthealth.com/blog/weight-man
   agement/9-health-benefits-of-weight-loss

7. 35 Surprising Benefits of Weight Loss

   https://doctormarvin.com/benefits-of-weight-loss
   /35-surprising-benefits-weight-loss/

8. 7 Important Health Benefits of Losing Weight

   https://www.hstinleypark.com/blog/7-important-h
   ealth-benefits-of-losing-weight

9. Top 12 Biggest Myths About Weight Loss

   https://www.healthline.com/nutrition/top-12-bigg
   est-myths-about-weight-loss

10.　How to naturally lose weight fast
https://www.medicalnewstoday.com/articles/322
345#fiber

11.　Benefits of maintaining weight loss
https://www.hopkinsmedicine.org/health/wellnes
s-and-prevention/maintaining-weight-loss

12.　14 weight-loss mistakes and how to avoid
them
https://www.weightwatchers.com/us/blog/weight
-loss/weight-loss-struggles

ABOUT THE AUTHOR

Charity Sago is a lover of books and a growth-enthusiast. She also enjoys giving out love via volunteer services.

As a person who is passionate about living a fulfilling life, she believes that a healthy person can achieve such desire. This led her to write Fit to Fly, a guide to healthy weight loss.